D0885436

MANIFEST DESTINY

JOURNAL

JUSTIN CARSON

Copyright © 2021 by Winterwolf Press. All rights reserved.

This book or any portion thereof may not be reproduced or used in any manner whatsoever without the express written permission from the publisher except for the use of brief quotations in critical articles, reviews, and pages where permission is specifically granted by the publisher.

First Edition

ISBN: 978-0-578-93458-7

Although the author and publisher have made every effort to ensure that the information in this book was correct at press time, the author and publisher do not assume and hereby disclaim any liability to any party for any loss, damage, or disruption caused by errors or omissions, whether such errors or omissions result from negligence, accident, or any other cause. Likewise, the author and publisher assume no responsibility for any false information. No liability is assumed for damages that may result from the reading or use of information contained within. The author has been told that this book contains highly emotional material regarding life and death, and that it challenges core belief systems. Read at your own risk. The views of this publication do not necessarily reflect the views of Winterwolf Press.

Books may be purchased by contacting the publisher at:

Chapter and Cover art by José Suárez

CONTENTS

FOREWORD

START MANIFESTING ANYTHING YOU WANT WITH THIS AMAZING MAGICAL MANIFESTING JOURNAL BY JUSTIN CARSON

If manifesting is your goal, then this Manifestation Journal by Justin Carson will be a great tool! It helps you manifest anything from destiny to manifesting more money. The journal directs you in several areas of manifesting: Goals, Progress, and Reflections. Justin Carson teaches you to create a list of what you want to manifest in each category (love, money, etc.). Every day, write down how far you are towards manifesting that goal. When you do this process for thirty days straight, without missing any days or skipping ahead - something amazing happens! You'll notice major changes in your life as your goals start showing up.

It is interesting how hard it can sometimes be for us to manifest things into our lives. Sometimes, an opportunity may seem like a good idea when you first think about it and later realize potential issues lurking behind your decision. Instead of jumping all in, take the time to consider all aspects. Justin Carson's manifestation journal helps to guide you in the right direction.

There are many different 'definitions' of the word manifest, but the simplest would be that a manifestation is 'something that is put into your physical reality through thought, feelings, and beliefs'.

This means that whatever you focus on is what you are bringing into your reality. You may focus and manifest through meditation, visualization, or just via your conscious or subconscious.

This manifestation journal will help you create and manifest your destiny. What you focus on manifesting is brought into your life or reality. You may not think that it's possible, but I promise this has helped me with my own manifestation journey!

Some people can manifest in their sleep because they don't have the conscious mind blocking them from seeing the outcome of their wishes before they're allowed to manifest them...some people rewrite history by changing recent events after feeling as if something should have happened differently. This Manifesting Journal will help you create the reality you desire.

If you can start working on believing, then there won't be anything holding back your manifestations!! Use this journal and believe in yourself!!!

Billy Carson
   4biddenknowledge Inc
   4biddenknowledge.com
   4biddenknowledge.tv
   UniteThe99.com

GRAB YOUR FREE 4BIDDENKNOWLEDGE TRIAL!

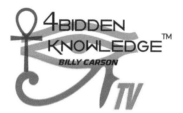

4biddenknowledge.com

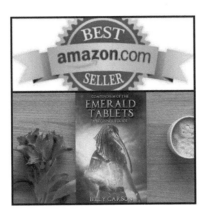

Billy Carson, the founder of <u>4biddenknowledge</u> Inc. Billy Carson is the Author of 'The Compendium Of The Emerald Tablets' and is an expert host on Deep Space, an original streaming series by Gaia.

The history of the Emerald Tablets is strange and beyond the belief of modern scientists. Their antiquity is stupendous, dating back some 36,000 years B.C. The author is Thoth, an Atlantean Priest-King who founded a colony in ancient Egypt, wrote the Emerald Tablets in his native Atlantean language which was translated by many famous scholars. This compendium of the Emerald Tablets gives unique insight and understanding of the content. Billy Carson breaks down each tablet for the reader. Because of the tablet's reference to the Egypt and sacred geometry they became a priority reference for those studying the Flower of Life and the Merkaba meditation. ORDER NOW.

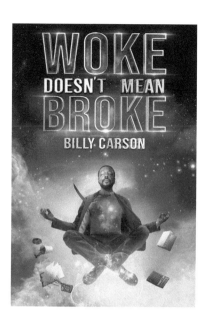

This is truly the time to make changes. Do not wait for anything or anybody. Now is the time to make your move. You need to be ahead of the game with the right tools that this book will provide you on your journey into the future. BUY NOW.

MANIFEST DESTINY

JOURNAL

By Author Justin Carson

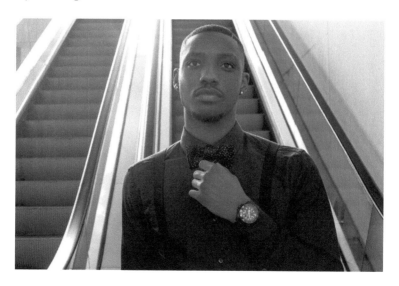

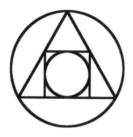

"WHAT EXISTS PHYSICALLY EXISTS FIRST IN THOUGHT AND FEELING. THERE IS NO OTHER RULE."

Jane Roberts

THE HERMETIC PRINCIPLE OF MENTALISM

"The **ALL** is **MIND**. The **Universe** is **Mental**".

TO START MANIFESTING YOUR REALITY, you must first understand that you are **one** with the **creator** thus giving you the ability to create. Human beings are creators and we have manifested everything you see here are Earth. Our thoughts lead to the manifestation of things and events. Everything in your reality is a manifestation of your mind. What you think and how you believe reality to work is true to you. Once you change your mind you can change the way you look at reality and reality will change. Our thoughts create our state of existence and the quality of our experience here on Earth. Therefore, be **responsible** for everything you create by being responsible for everything that you **think.**

THE HERMETIC PRINCIPLE OF CORRESPONDENCE

"As ABOVE, so below; As below, so above".

The outer world is nothing more than a reflection of our inner world. How you believe reality to work, and what you believe to be possible or impossible is reflected in the external world. If you have fears, doubts, and indecision within, it will be created and reflected in your outer world as fears, doubts, and indecision. If you operate from a place of decisiveness, and unwavering faith and conviction in your ability to create and manifest, that's when you will start to see change.

What you put out into the universe is what you will receive back and it works both positively and negatively. Have you ever met a person that every time you talk to them they always have something negative to say, they complain about everything, and always have some type of drama going on? This is just a reflection of what they have going on within themselves. The more you speak negatively about yourself or other people, the more negativity you'll attract, and the more you complain the universe is just going to giving you more things to complain about. With that being said always operate form a mindset of Positivity, Abundance, Gratefulness, optimism, and Power and that's what you will attract into your life.

THE POWER OF I AM

"I AM... two of the most powerful words; for what you put after them shapes your reality".

— BEVAN LEE

"I AM" is the most powerful command statement there is. The power to create your own reality is already in you because you are **GOD** and **GOD** is you, you are the "**Source Energy**". The divine energy that makes up this entire universe is inside of you and because of this divinity; you have the power of creation. I AM can be used to empower or disempower you, so be careful of what you attach to the end of that statement; it will manifest into reality. In fact, you are already speaking it into your life. When you say negative things like I'm frustrated, I'm overwhelmed, I'm not good enough, you're in essence saying I AM and this negativity will put you in a state of low vibration and you will just keep attracting more negativity. When you say I'm grateful, I'm able, and highly favored, you're also saying "I AM"! Change the way you view and talk to yourself because your subconscious mind is always listening.

THE STEPS TO MANIFESTING YOUR DESTINY

EVERY DAY you are going to write down 3 things you are grateful for. Life is a continuous cycle of giving and receiving energy. Be thankful for who and what you have already in your life, instead of complaining about what you don't have. When you express gratitude it automatically raises your vibration, which will allow you to attract prosperity and abundance. Next you will write down what you are trying to manifest in detail. For example if you are trying to manifest a car write down the make, model, what color do you want it to be, will it be a two door or four door, how much money you need to put down, every little detail you can think of, then take a minute to close your eyes and visualize yourself already having it. You can even go to the dealership to look at the car, sit in it, and test drive the car is they let you. After you have written down what you want to manifest (In detail) write down what actions you are going to take to attract it.

"Things may come to those who wait, but only the thing left by those who hustle" −Abraham Lincoln. You must take action on what you're trying to manifest. So whatever it is that's going to get you closer to what you want you go out and do it, even if doubts and fears creep into your thoughts. Don't be afraid to fail, a lot of people have missed out on their true calling because of fear and instead of pushing past that initial fear of the unknown they chose to not take action. You will not be one of those people who didn't take action, you are bigger than you fears, and if you fail, brush it off, learn from your mistakes and prepare yourself for the next opportunity presented to you. Lastly you will write down 10 positive affirmations about yourself preceded by the words "I AM" speaking them aloud as you go. Remember the more you write, speak, and visualize your manifestation the quicker it will become a reality. Always remember to spread peace and love throughout the world and to be the light among darkness.

I AM THE UNIVERSE AND THE UNIVERSE IS ME

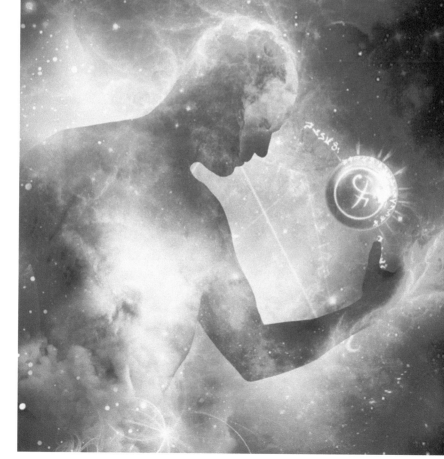

Date:_____ / _____ / _____

What are three things you're grateful for?

1. _____

2. _____

3. _____

What are you manifesting and what actions will

you take to attract it?

_____

_____

_____

_____

_____

_____

Write down 10 positive affirmations
About yourself
(Speak out loud)

1. I AM_____

2. I AM_____

3. I AM_____

4. I AM_____

5. I AM_____

6. I AM_____

7. I AM_____

8. I AM_____

9. I AM_____

10. I AM_____

I AM THE CREATOR OF MY REALITY

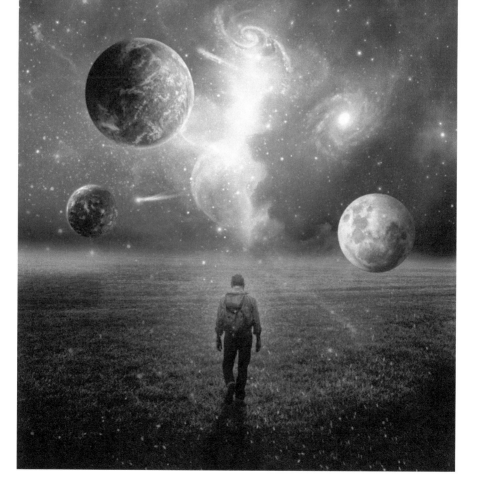

Date:_____ / _____ / _____

What are three things you're grateful for?

1. _____

2. _____

3. _____

What are you manifesting and what actions will you take to attract it?

_____

_____

_____

_____

_____

_____

Write down 10 positive affirmations
About yourself
(Speak out loud)

1. I AM_____

2. I AM_____

3. I AM_____

4. I AM_____

5. I AM_____

6. I AM_____

7. I AM_____

8. I AM_____

9. I AM_____

10. I AM_____

I AM UNDER UNIVERSAL GUIDANCE AND PROTECTION

I AM UNDER UNIVERSAL GUIDANCE & PROTECTION

Date:____ / ____ / ____

What are three things you're grateful for?

1. _____

2. _____

3. _____

What are you manifesting and what actions will you take to attract it?

_____

_____

_____

_____

_____

_____

Write down 10 positive affirmations
About yourself
(Speak out loud)

1. I AM_____

2. I AM_____

3. I AM_____

4. I AM_____

5. I AM_____

6. I AM_____

7. I AM_____

8. I AM_____

9. I AM_____

10. I AM_____

8

I AM ONE WITH THE CREATOR AND
THE CREATOR IS ONE WITH ME

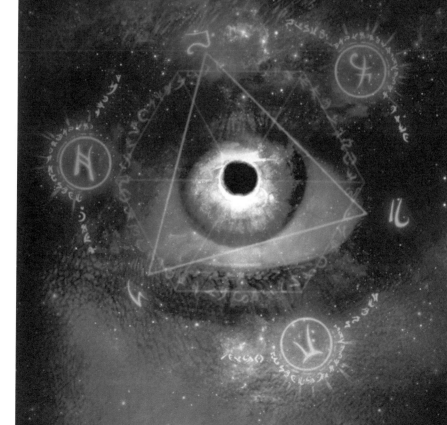

Date:____ / ____ / ____

What are three things you're grateful for?

1. _____

2. _____

3. _____

What are you manifesting and what actions will

you take to attract it?

_____

_____

_____

_____

_____

_____

Write down 10 positive affirmations
About yourself
(Speak out loud)

1. I AM_____

2. I AM_____

3. I AM_____

4. I AM_____

5. I AM_____

6. I AM_____

7. I AM_____

8. I AM_____

9. I AM_____

10. I AM_____

9

I AM LIVING IN ABUNDANCE

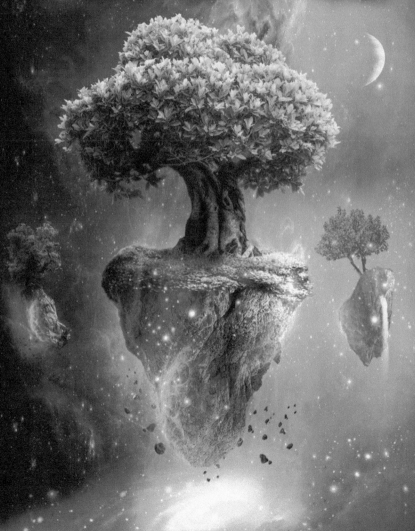

I AM LIVING IN ABUNDANCE

Date:_____ / _____ / _____

What are three things you're grateful for?

1. _____

2. _____

3. _____

What are you manifesting and what actions will you take to attract it?

_____

_____

_____

_____

_____

_____

Write down 10 positive affirmations
About yourself
(Speak out loud)

1. I AM_____

2. I AM_____

3. I AM_____

4. I AM_____

5. I AM_____

6. I AM_____

7. I AM_____

8. I AM_____

9. I AM_____

10. I AM_____

I AM BIGGER THAN MY FEARS

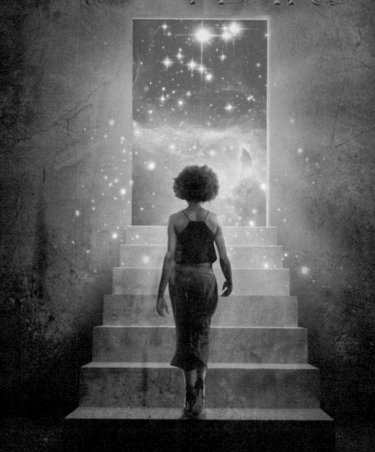

Date:_____ / _____ / _____

What are three things you're grateful for?

1. _____

2. _____

3. _____

What are you manifesting and what actions will

you take to attract it?

_____

_____

_____

_____

_____

_____

Write down 10 positive affirmations
About yourself
(Speak out loud)

1. I AM_____

2. I AM_____

3. I AM_____

4. I AM_____

5. I AM_____

6. I AM_____

7. I AM_____

8. I AM_____

9. I AM_____

10. I AM_____

11

I AM THE SOURCE ENERGY

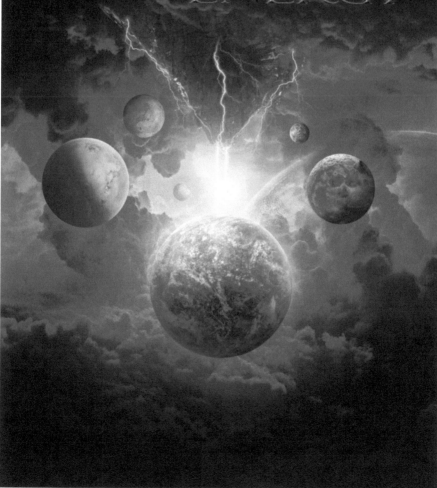

Date:____ / ____ / ____

What are three things you're grateful for?

1. _____

2. _____

3. _____

What are you manifesting and what actions will

you take to attract it?

_____

_____

_____

_____

_____

_____

Write down 10 positive affirmations
About yourself
(Speak out loud)

1. I AM_____

2. I AM_____

3. I AM_____

4. I AM_____

5. I AM_____

6. I AM_____

7. I AM_____

8. I AM_____

9. I AM_____

10. I AM_____

12

I AM LIVING MY DREAM LIFE

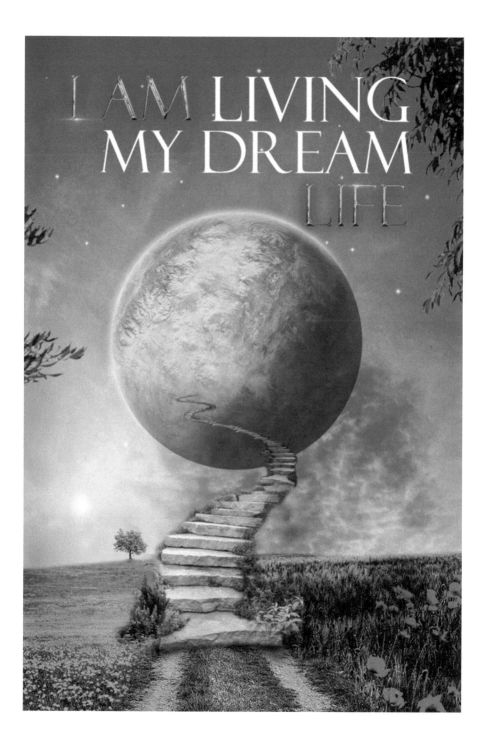

Date:_____ / _____ / _____

What are three things you're grateful for?

1. _____

2. _____

3. _____

What are you manifesting and what actions will you take to attract it?

_____

_____

_____

_____

_____

_____

Write down 10 positive affirmations
About yourself
(Speak out loud)

1. I AM_____

2. I AM_____

3. I AM_____

4. I AM_____

5. I AM_____

6. I AM_____

7. I AM_____

8. I AM_____

9. I AM_____

10. I AM_____

13

I AM A MAGNET FOR MIRACLES

I AM A MAGNET FOR MIRACLES

Date:____ / ____ / ____

What are three things you're grateful for?

1. _____

2. _____

3. _____

What are you manifesting and what actions will you take to attract it?

_____

_____

_____

_____

_____

_____

Write down 10 positive affirmations
About yourself
(Speak out loud)

1. I AM_____

2. I AM_____

3. I AM_____

4. I AM_____

5. I AM_____

6. I AM_____

7. I AM_____

8. I AM_____

9. I AM_____

10. I AM_____

14

I AM FREE FROM ALL STRESS AND ANXIETY

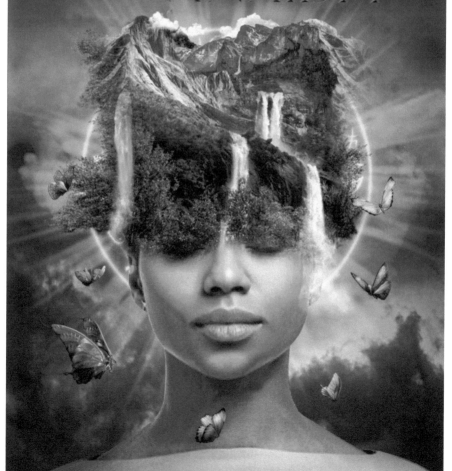

I AM FREE FROM ALL STRESS & ANXIETY

Date:____ / ____ / ____

What are three things you're grateful for?

1. _____

2. _____

3. _____

What are you manifesting and what actions will you take to attract it?

_____

_____

_____

_____

_____

_____

Write down 10 positive affirmations
About yourself
(Speak out loud)

1. I AM_____

2. I AM_____

3. I AM_____

4. I AM_____

5. I AM_____

6. I AM_____

7. I AM_____

8. I AM_____

9. I AM_____

10. I AM_____

15

I AM AT PEACE WITH MY PAST

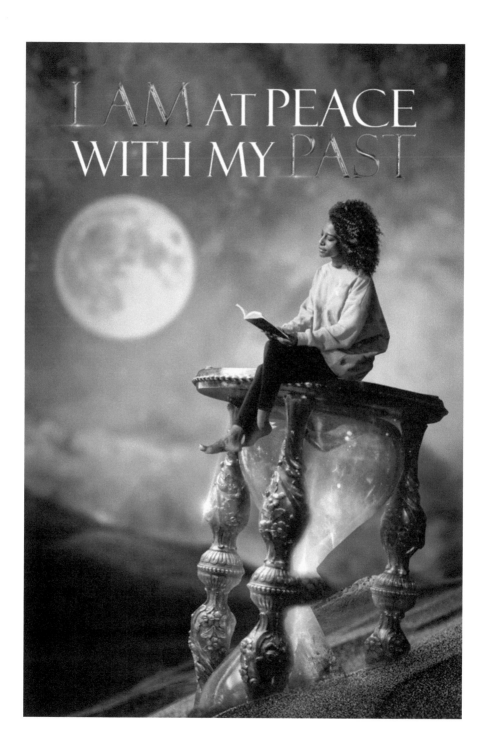

Date:____ / ____ / ____

What are three things you're grateful for?

1. _____

2. _____

3. _____

What are you manifesting and what actions will you take to attract it?

_____

_____

_____

_____

_____

_____

Write down 10 positive affirmations
About yourself
(Speak out loud)

1. I AM_____

2. I AM_____

3. I AM_____

4. I AM_____

5. I AM_____

6. I AM_____

7. I AM_____

8. I AM_____

9. I AM_____

10. I AM_____

16

I AM THE ARCHITECT OF MY LIFE

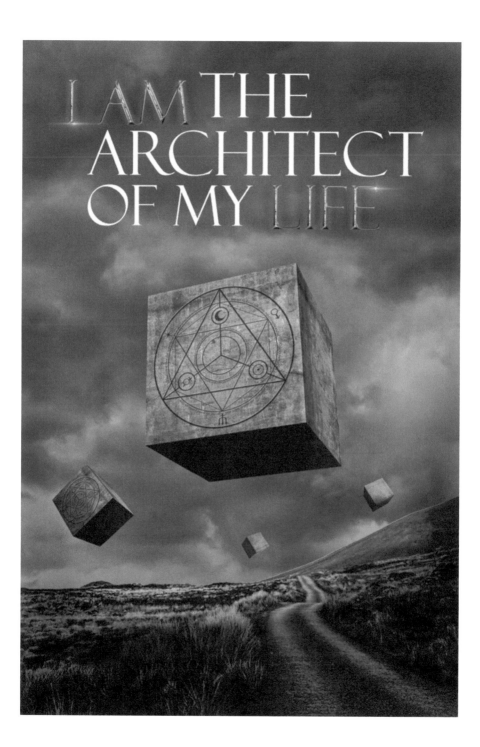

Date:____ / ____ / ____

What are three things you're grateful for?

1. _____

2. _____

3. _____

What are you manifesting and what actions will you take to attract it?

_____

_____

_____

_____

_____

_____

Write down 10 positive affirmations
About yourself
(Speak out loud)

1. I AM_____

2. I AM_____

3. I AM_____

4. I AM_____

5. I AM_____

6. I AM_____

7. I AM_____

8. I AM_____

9. I AM_____

10. I AM_____

17

I AM CONFIDENT IN MY ABILITY TO MANIFEST

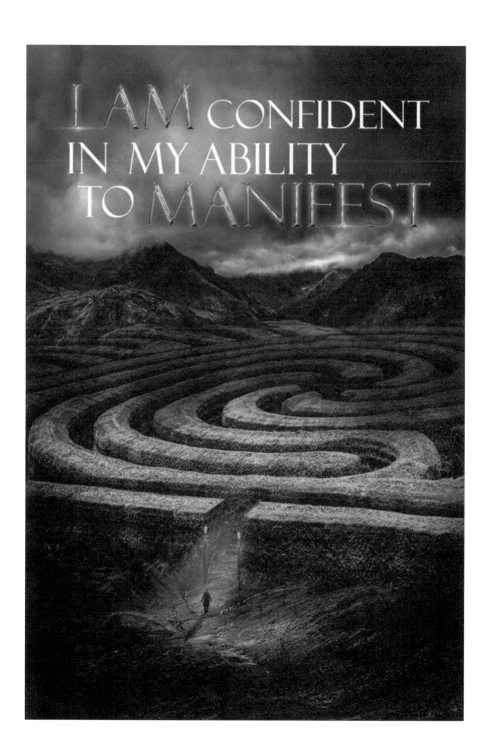

Date:____ / ____ / ____

What are three things you're grateful for?

1. _____

2. _____

3. _____

What are you manifesting and what actions will you take to attract it?

_____

_____

_____

_____

_____

_____

Write down 10 positive affirmations
About yourself
(Speak out loud)

1. I AM_____

2. I AM_____

3. I AM_____

4. I AM_____

5. I AM_____

6. I AM_____

7. I AM_____

8. I AM_____

9. I AM_____

10. I AM_____

18

I AM IN COMPLETE CONTROL OF MY LIFE

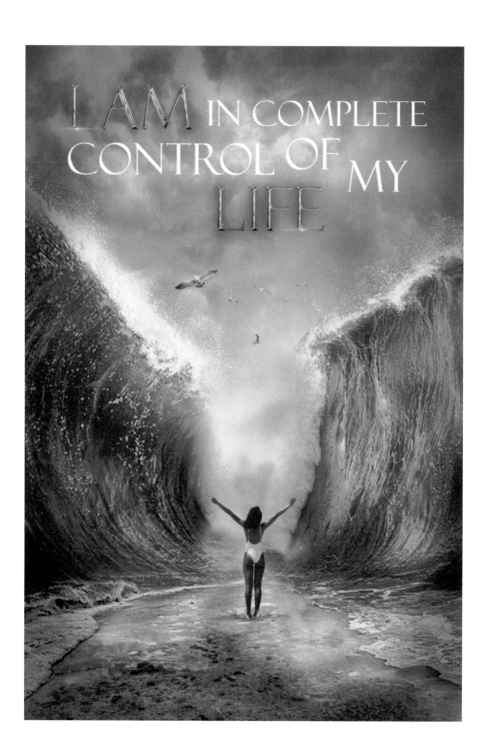

Date:_____ / _____ / _____

What are three things you're grateful for?

1. _____

2. _____

3. _____

What are you manifesting and what actions will you take to attract it?

_____

_____

_____

_____

_____

_____

Write down 10 positive affirmations
About yourself
(Speak out loud)

1. I AM_____

2. I AM_____

3. I AM_____

4. I AM_____

5. I AM_____

6. I AM_____

7. I AM_____

8. I AM_____

9. I AM_____

10. I AM_____

19

I AM A CONSCIOUS CREATOR

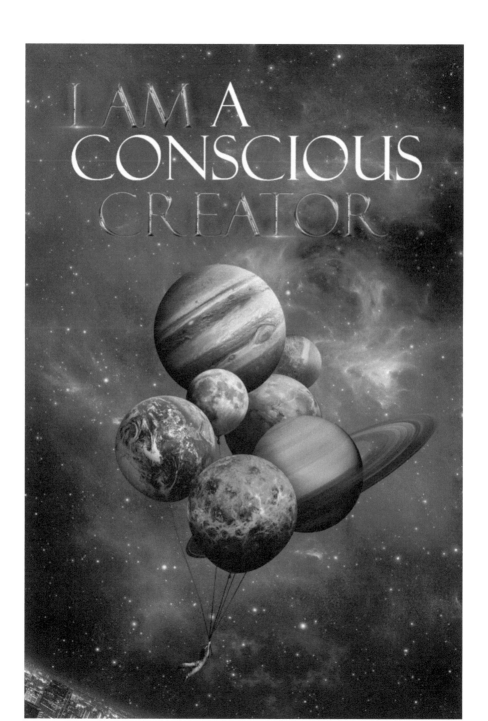

Date:_____ / _____ / _____

What are three things you're grateful for?

1. _____

2. _____

3. _____

What are you manifesting and what actions will you take to attract it?

_____

_____

_____

_____

_____

_____

Write down 10 positive affirmations
About yourself
(Speak out loud)

1. I AM_____

2. I AM_____

3. I AM_____

4. I AM_____

5. I AM_____

6. I AM_____

7. I AM_____

8. I AM_____

9. I AM_____

10. I AM_____

20

I AM CREATING MY OWN DESTINY

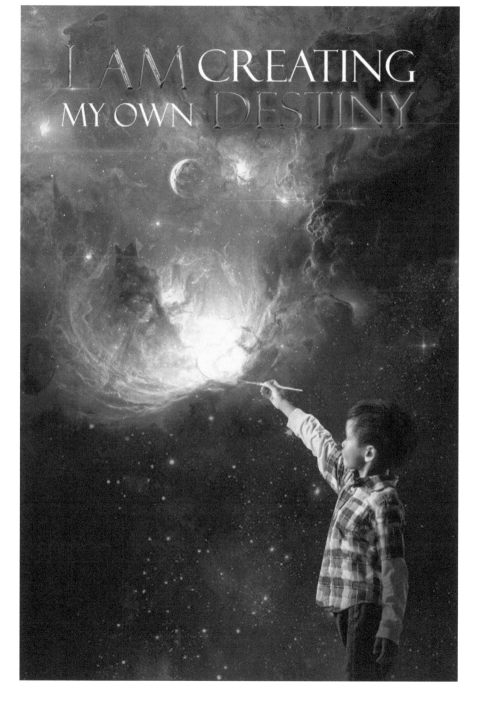

Date:____ / ____ / ____

What are three things you're grateful for?

1. _____

2. _____

3. _____

What are you manifesting and what actions will

you take to attract it?

_____

_____

_____

_____

_____

_____

Write down 10 positive affirmations
About yourself
(Speak out loud)

1. I AM_____

2. I AM_____

3. I AM_____

4. I AM_____

5. I AM_____

6. I AM_____

7. I AM_____

8. I AM_____

9. I AM_____

10. I AM_____

21

I AM CREATING MY OWN SUCCESS

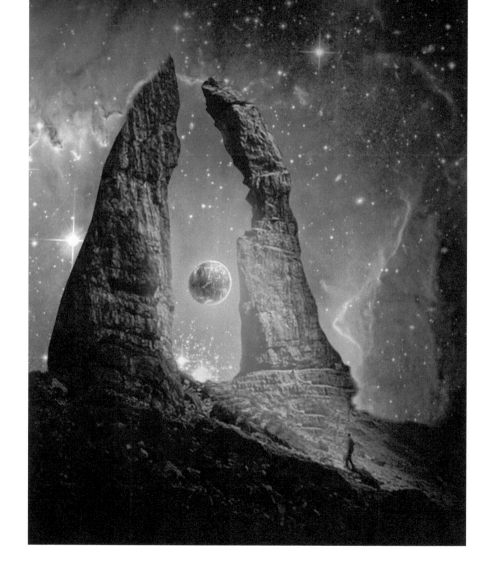

Date:_____ / _____ / _____

What are three things you're grateful for?

1. _____

2. _____

3. _____

What are you manifesting and what actions will

you take to attract it?

_____

_____

_____

_____

_____

_____

Write down 10 positive affirmations
About yourself
(Speak out loud)

1. I AM_____

2. I AM_____

3. I AM_____

4. I AM_____

5. I AM_____

6. I AM_____

7. I AM_____

8. I AM_____

9. I AM_____

10. I AM_____

22

I AM WORTHY AND DESERVING OF SUCCESS

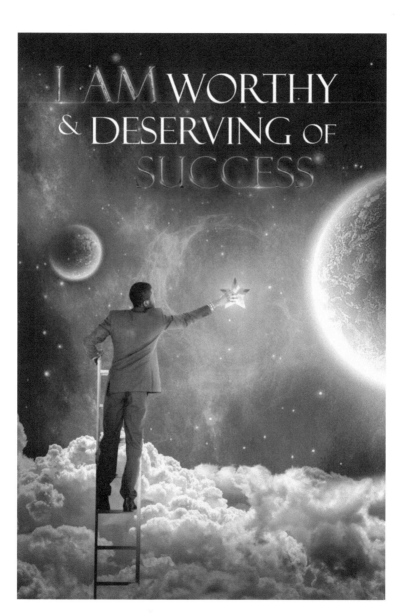

Date:_____ / _____ / _____

What are three things you're grateful for?

1. _____

2. _____

3. _____

What are you manifesting and what actions will

you take to attract it?

_____

_____

_____

_____

_____

_____

Write down 10 positive affirmations
About yourself
(Speak out loud)

1. I AM_____

2. I AM_____

3. I AM_____

4. I AM_____

5. I AM_____

6. I AM_____

7. I AM_____

8. I AM_____

9. I AM_____

10. I AM_____

I AM NOT AFRAID TO FAIL

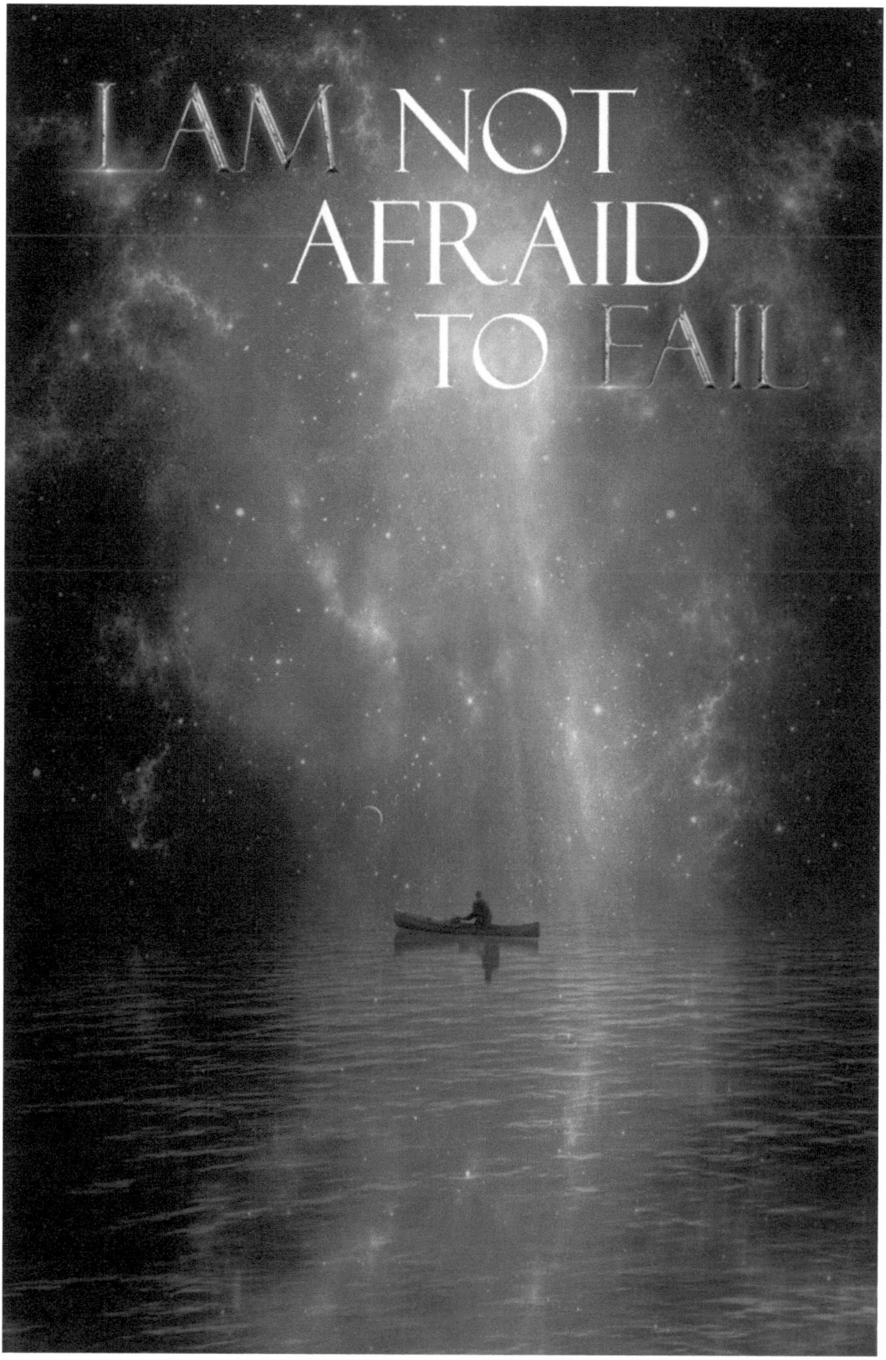
I AM NOT
AFRAID
TO FAIL

Date:_____ / _____ / _____

What are three things you're grateful for?

1. _____

2. _____

3. _____

What are you manifesting and what actions will

you take to attract it?

_____

_____

_____

_____

_____

_____

Write down 10 positive affirmations
About yourself
(Speak out loud)

1. I AM_____

2. I AM_____

3. I AM_____

4. I AM_____

5. I AM_____

6. I AM_____

7. I AM_____

8. I AM_____

9. I AM_____

10. I AM_____

24

I AM IMPORTANT

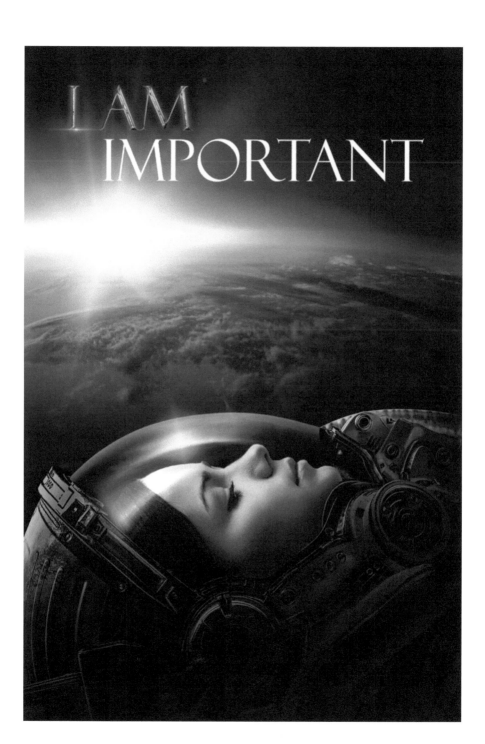

Date:____ / ____ / ____

What are three things you're grateful for?

1. _____

2. _____

3. _____

What are you manifesting and what actions will you take to attract it?

_____

_____

_____

_____

_____

Write down 10 positive affirmations
About yourself
(Speak out loud)

1. I AM_____

2. I AM_____

3. I AM_____

4. I AM_____

5. I AM_____

6. I AM_____

7. I AM_____

8. I AM_____

9. I AM_____

10. I AM_____

25

I AM PROUD OF MYSELF

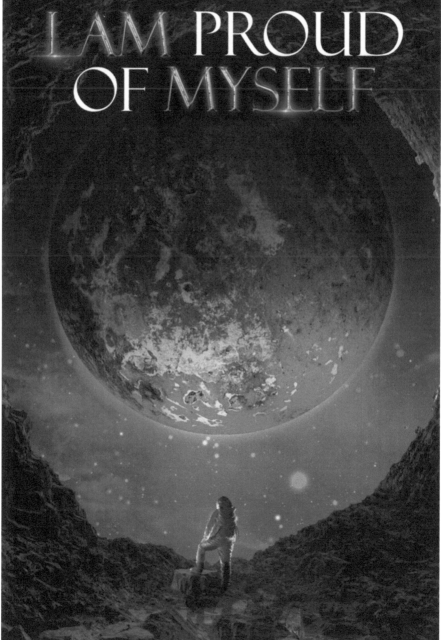

Date:____ / ____ / ____

What are three things you're grateful for?

1. _____

2. _____

3. _____

What are you manifesting and what actions will you take to attract it?

_____

_____

_____

_____

_____

_____

Write down 10 positive affirmations
About yourself
(Speak out loud)

1. I AM_____

2. I AM_____

3. I AM_____

4. I AM_____

5. I AM_____

6. I AM_____

7. I AM_____

8. I AM_____

9. I AM_____

10. I AM_____

26

I AM ONE OF A KIND

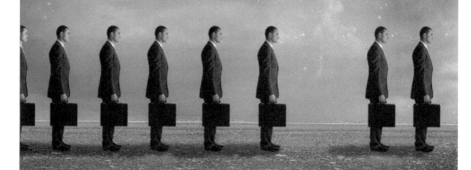

Date:_____ / _____ / _____

What are three things you're grateful for?

1. _____

2. _____

3. _____

What are you manifesting and what actions will you take to attract it?

_____

_____

_____

_____

_____

_____

Write down 10 positive affirmations
About yourself
(Speak out loud)

1. I AM_____

2. I AM_____

3. I AM_____

4. I AM_____

5. I AM_____

6. I AM_____

7. I AM_____

8. I AM_____

9. I AM_____

10. I AM_____

27

I AM TRUSTING THE TIMING OF MY LIFE

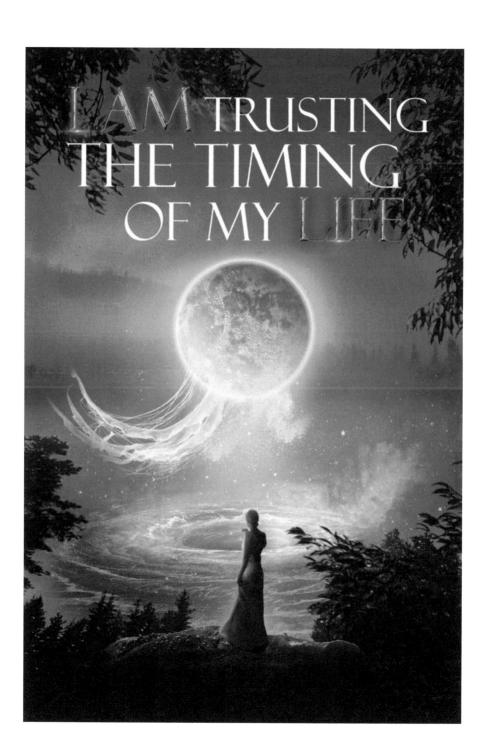

I AM TRUSTING
THE TIMING
OF MY LIFE

Date:_____ / _____ / _____

What are three things you're grateful for?

1. _____

2. _____

3. _____

What are you manifesting and what actions will you take to attract it?

_____

_____

_____

_____

_____

_____

Write down 10 positive affirmations
About yourself
(Speak out loud)

1. I AM_____

2. I AM_____

3. I AM_____

4. I AM_____

5. I AM_____

6. I AM_____

7. I AM_____

8. I AM_____

9. I AM_____

10. I AM_____

28

I AM NOT AFRIAD TO SUCCEED

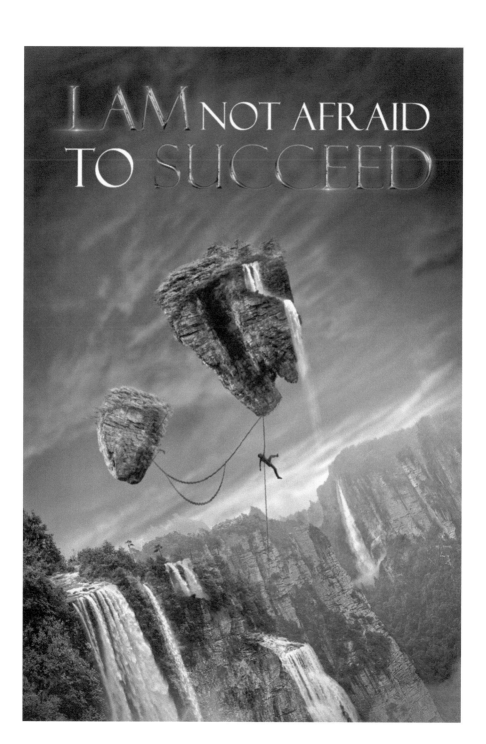

Date:_____ / _____ / _____

What are three things you're grateful for?

1. _____

2. _____

3. _____

What are you manifesting and what actions will you take to attract it?

_____

_____

_____

_____

_____

_____

Write down 10 positive affirmations
About yourself
(Speak out loud)

1. I AM_____

2. I AM_____

3. I AM_____

4. I AM_____

5. I AM_____

6. I AM_____

7. I AM_____

8. I AM_____

9. I AM_____

10. I AM_____

29

I AM DIFFERENT AND THAT'S OKAY

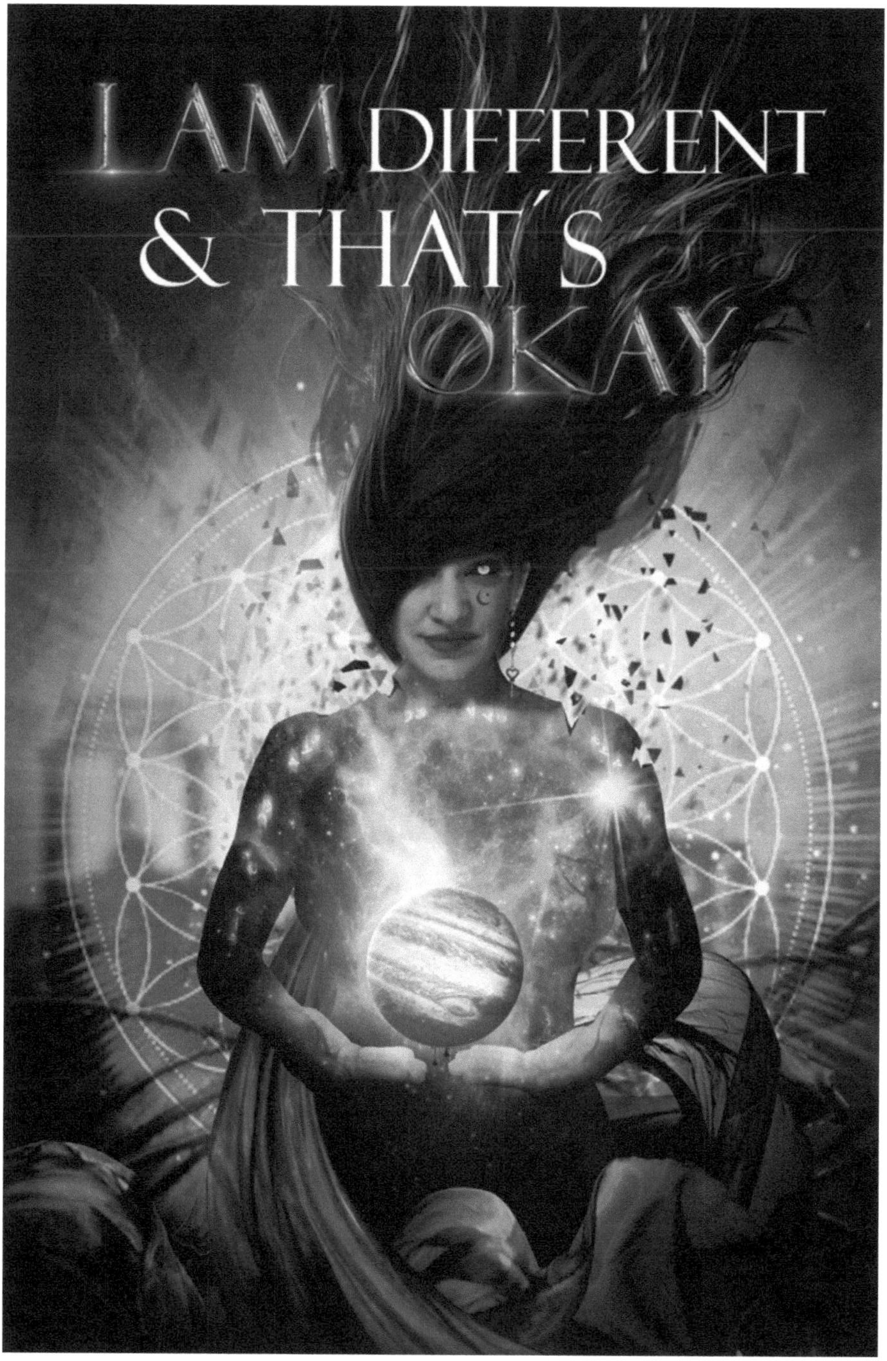
I AM DIFFERENT
& THAT´S
OKAY

Date:_____ / _____ / _____

What are three things you're grateful for?

1. _____

2. _____

3. _____

What are you manifesting and what actions will

you take to attract it?

_____

_____

_____

_____

_____

_____

Write down 10 positive affirmations
About yourself
(Speak out loud)

1. I AM_____

2. I AM_____

3. I AM_____

4. I AM_____

5. I AM_____

6. I AM_____

7. I AM_____

8. I AM_____

9. I AM_____

10. I AM_____

30

I AM READY FOR WHATEVER LIFE
THROWS AT ME

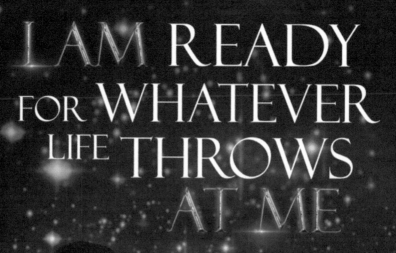

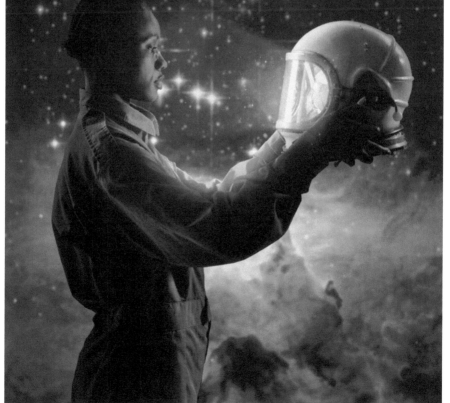

Date:____ / ____ / ____

What are three things you're grateful for?

1. _____

2. _____

3. _____

What are you manifesting and what actions will you take to attract it?

_____

_____

_____

_____

_____

_____

Write down 10 positive affirmations
About yourself
(Speak out loud)

1. I AM_____

2. I AM_____

3. I AM_____

4. I AM_____

5. I AM_____

6. I AM_____

7. I AM_____

8. I AM_____

9. I AM_____

10. I AM_____

31

I AM LIVING THE LIFE I WANT

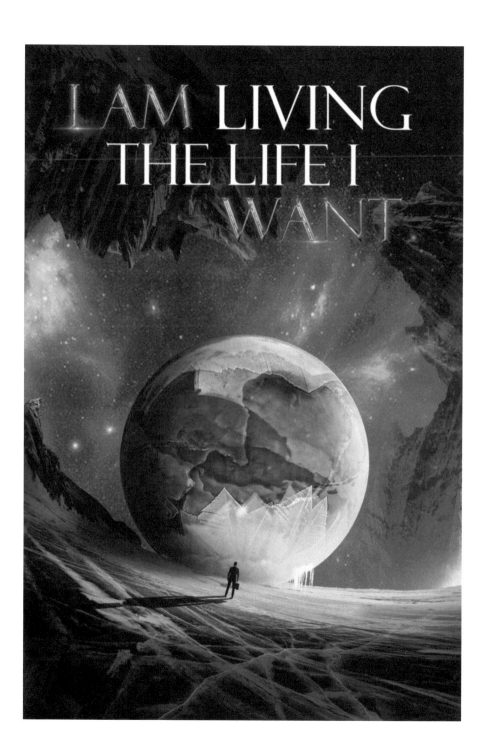

Date:____ / ____ / ____

What are three things you're grateful for?

1. _____

2. _____

3. _____

What are you manifesting and what actions will you take to attract it?

_____

_____

_____

_____

_____

_____

Write down 10 positive affirmations
About yourself
(Speak out loud)

1. I AM_____

2. I AM_____

3. I AM_____

4. I AM_____

5. I AM_____

6. I AM_____

7. I AM_____

8. I AM_____

9. I AM_____

10. I AM_____

32

I AM ATTRACTING WEALTH AND
PROSPERTY

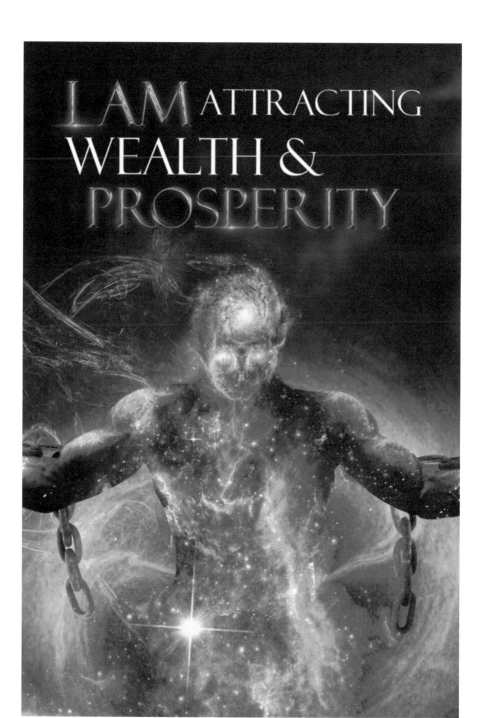

Date:____ / ____ / ____

What are three things you're grateful for?

1. _____

2. _____

3. _____

What are you manifesting and what actions will you take to attract it?

_____

_____

_____

_____

_____

_____

Write down 10 positive affirmations
About yourself
(Speak out loud)

1. I AM_____

2. I AM_____

3. I AM_____

4. I AM_____

5. I AM_____

6. I AM_____

7. I AM_____

8. I AM_____

9. I AM_____

10. I AM_____

33

I AM A MAGNET FOR MONEY

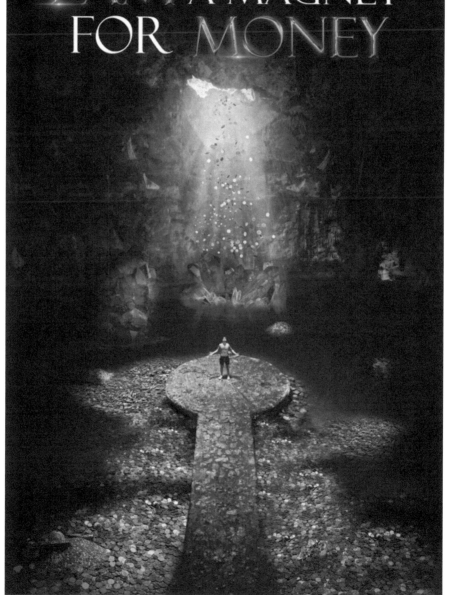

Date:____ / ____ / ____

What are three things you're grateful for?

1. _____

2. _____

3. _____

What are you manifesting and what actions will

you take to attract it?

_____

_____

_____

_____

_____

_____

Write down 10 positive affirmations
About yourself
(Speak out loud)

1. I AM_____

2. I AM_____

3. I AM_____

4. I AM_____

5. I AM_____

6. I AM_____

7. I AM_____

8. I AM_____

9. I AM_____

10. I AM_____

34

I AM PROUD OF WHO I AM AND WHO
I AM BECOMING

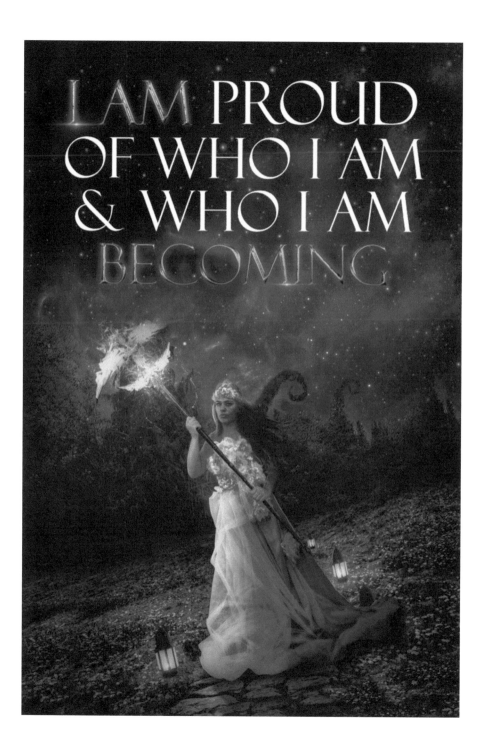

Date:_____ / _____ / _____

What are three things you're grateful for?

1. _____

2. _____

3. _____

What are you manifesting and what actions will you take to attract it?

_____

_____

_____

_____

_____

_____

Write down 10 positive affirmations
About yourself
(Speak out loud)

1. I AM_____

2. I AM_____

3. I AM_____

4. I AM_____

5. I AM_____

6. I AM_____

7. I AM_____

8. I AM_____

9. I AM_____

10. I AM_____

35

I AM HIGHLY FAVORED BY THE UNIVERSE

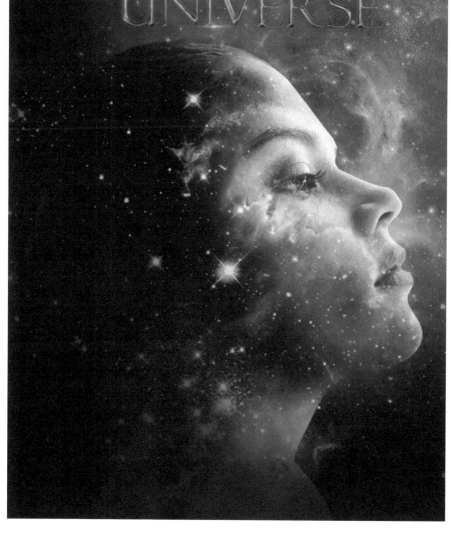

Date:____ / ____ / ____

What are three things you're grateful for?

1. _____

2. _____

3. _____

What are you manifesting and what actions will

you take to attract it?

_____

_____

_____

_____

_____

_____

Write down 10 positive affirmations
About yourself
(Speak out loud)

1. I AM_____

2. I AM_____

3. I AM_____

4. I AM_____

5. I AM_____

6. I AM_____

7. I AM_____

8. I AM_____

9. I AM_____

10. I AM_____

36

I AM WANTED AND LOVED

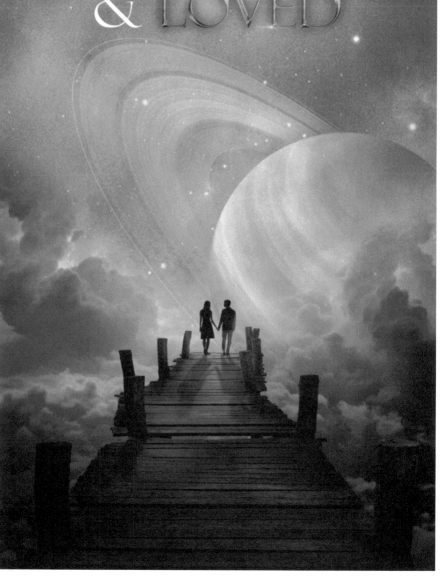

Date:_____ / _____ / _____

What are three things you're grateful for?

1. _____

2. _____

3. _____

What are you manifesting and what actions will

you take to attract it?

_____

_____

_____

_____

_____

_____

Write down 10 positive affirmations
About yourself
(Speak out loud)

1. I AM_____

2. I AM_____

3. I AM_____

4. I AM_____

5. I AM_____

6. I AM_____

7. I AM_____

8. I AM_____

9. I AM_____

10. I AM_____

37

I AM IN CONTROL OF MY ACTIONS AND EMOTIONS

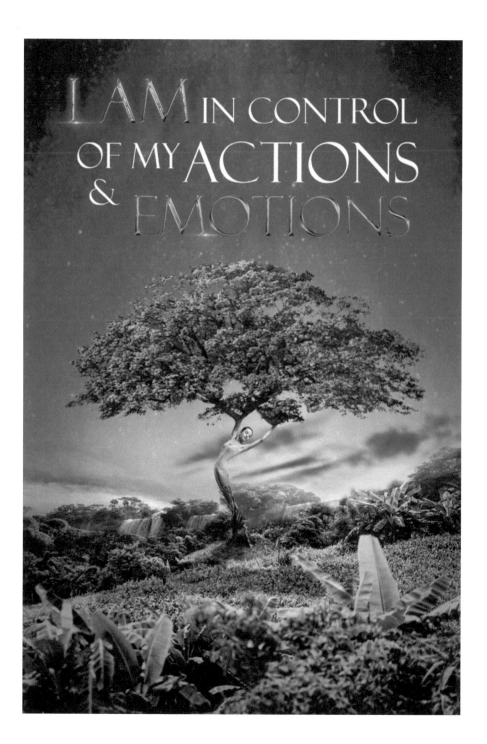

Date:____ / ____ / ____

What are three things you're grateful for?

1. _____

2. _____

3. _____

What are you manifesting and what actions will

you take to attract it?

_____

_____

_____

_____

_____

_____

Write down 10 positive affirmations
About yourself
(Speak out loud)

1. I AM_____

2. I AM_____

3. I AM_____

4. I AM_____

5. I AM_____

6. I AM_____

7. I AM_____

8. I AM_____

9. I AM_____

10. I AM_____

38

I AM FOCUSED ON ACHIEVING MY
GOALS

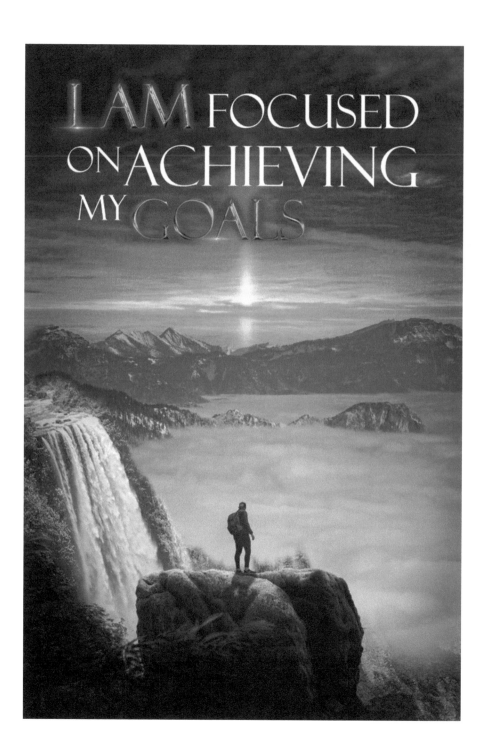

Date:____ / ____ / ____

What are three things you're grateful for?

1. _____

2. _____

3. _____

What are you manifesting and what actions will

you take to attract it?

_____

_____

_____

_____

_____

_____

Write down 10 positive affirmations
About yourself
(Speak out loud)

1. I AM_____

2. I AM_____

3. I AM_____

4. I AM_____

5. I AM_____

6. I AM_____

7. I AM_____

8. I AM_____

9. I AM_____

10. I AM_____

39

I AM BECOMING THE BEST VERSION OF MYSELF

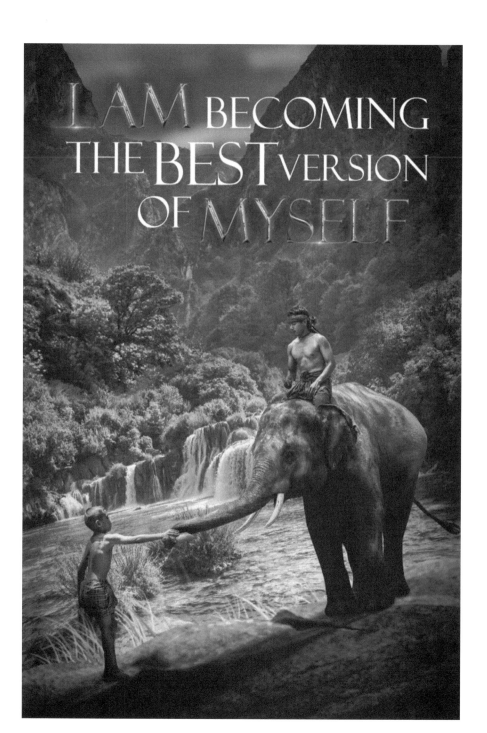

I AM BECOMING THE BEST VERSION OF MYSELF

Date:____ / ____ / ____

What are three things you're grateful for?

1. _____

2. _____

3. _____

What are you manifesting and what actions will

you take to attract it?

_____

_____

_____

_____

_____

_____

Write down 10 positive affirmations
About yourself
(Speak out loud)

1. I AM_____

2. I AM_____

3. I AM_____

4. I AM_____

5. I AM_____

6. I AM_____

7. I AM_____

8. I AM_____

9. I AM_____

10. I AM_____

40

I AM THE CHOSEN ONE

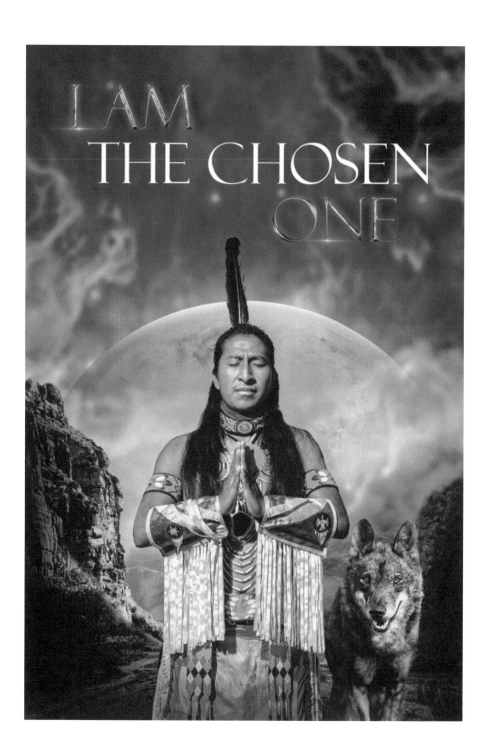

Date:____ / ____ / ____

What are three things you're grateful for?

1. _____

2. _____

3. _____

What are you manifesting and what actions will you take to attract it?

_____

_____

_____

_____

_____

_____

Write down 10 positive affirmations
About yourself
(Speak out loud)

1. I AM_____

2. I AM_____

3. I AM_____

4. I AM_____

5. I AM_____

6. I AM_____

7. I AM_____

8. I AM_____

9. I AM_____

10. I AM_____

41

I AM THE BEST VERSION OF MYSELF

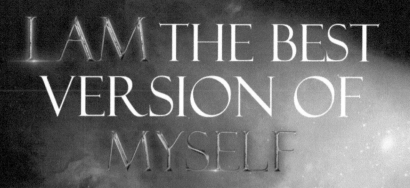

I AM THE BEST VERSION OF MYSELF

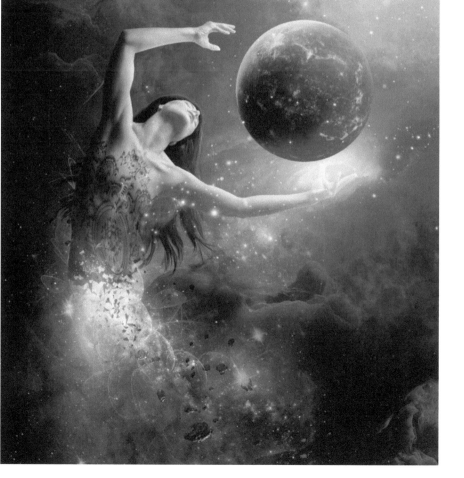

Date:_____ / _____ / _____

What are three things you're grateful for?

1. _____

2. _____

3. _____

What are you manifesting and what actions will

you take to attract it?

_____

_____

_____

_____

_____

_____

Write down 10 positive affirmations
About yourself
(Speak out loud)

1. I AM_____

2. I AM_____

3. I AM_____

4. I AM_____

5. I AM_____

6. I AM_____

7. I AM_____

8. I AM_____

9. I AM_____

10. I AM_____

42

I AM OVERFLOWING WITH JOY AND
HAPPINESS

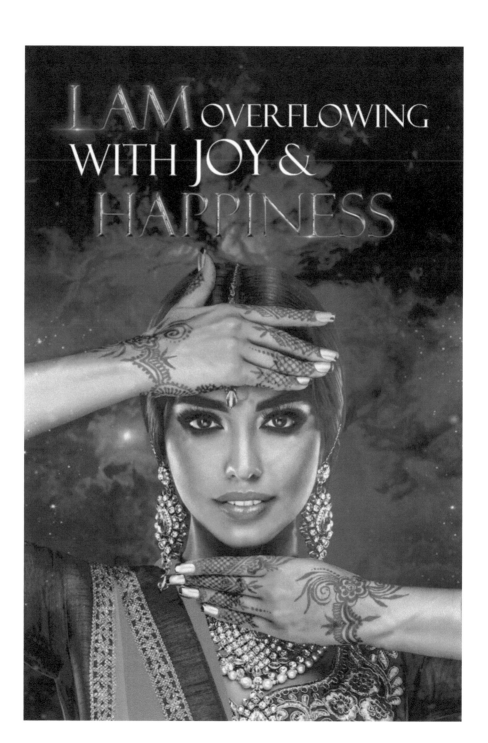

Date:_____ / _____ / _____

What are three things you're grateful for?

1. _____

2. _____

3. _____

What are you manifesting and what actions will

you take to attract it?

_____

_____

_____

_____

_____

_____

Write down 10 positive affirmations
About yourself
(Speak out loud)

1. I AM_____

2. I AM_____

3. I AM_____

4. I AM_____

5. I AM_____

6. I AM_____

7. I AM_____

8. I AM_____

9. I AM_____

10. I AM_____

43

WHAT HAVE YOU LEARNED ABOUT
YOURSELF

Date:____ / ____ / ____

What have you learned about yourself during this journey?

_____

_____

_____

_____

_____

_____

_____

_____

_____

_____

_____

_____

_____

_____

Date:____ / ____ / ____

Daily Diary

_____

_____

_____

_____

_____

_____

_____

_____

_____

_____

_____

_____

_____

_____

Date:____ / ____ / ____

Daily Diary

_____

_____

_____

_____

_____

_____

_____

_____

_____

_____

_____

_____

_____

_____

_____

Date:_____ / _____ / _____

Daily Diary

_____

_____

_____

_____

_____

_____

_____

_____

_____

_____

_____

_____

_____

_____

Date:____ / ____ / ____

Daily Diary

_____

_____

_____

_____

_____

_____

_____

_____

_____

_____

_____

_____

_____

_____

Date:_____ / _____ / _____

Daily Diary

_____

_____

_____

_____

_____

_____

_____

_____

_____

_____

_____

_____

_____

_____

_____

Date:_____ / _____ / _____

Daily Diary

_____

_____

_____

_____

_____

_____

_____

_____

_____

_____

_____

_____

_____

_____

Date:____ / ____ / ____

Daily Diary

_____

_____

_____

_____

_____

_____

_____

_____

_____

_____

_____

_____

_____

_____

_____

_____

Date:____ / ____ / ____

Daily Diary

_____

_____

_____

_____

_____

_____

_____

_____

_____

_____

_____

_____

_____

_____

Date:____ / ____ / ____

Daily Diary

_____

_____

_____

_____

_____

_____

_____

_____

_____

_____

_____

_____

_____

_____

_____

_____

Date:_____ / _____ / _____

Daily Diary

_____

_____

_____

_____

_____

_____

_____

_____

_____

_____

_____

_____

_____

_____